I0441264

Paleo Free Diet: Detox Diet:

Gluten Free Recipes & Wheat Free Recipes for Paleo Beginners; Detox Cleanse Diet to Lose Belly Fat & Increase Energy

Emma Rose

Paleo Free Diet Guide for Beginners

Over 50 Paleo Free Recipes for Optimal Health & Fast Weight Loss

Emma Rose

Image courtesy of rakratchada torsap / FreeDigitalPhotos.net

© Copyright 2014 by Joy Publishing & Marketing Corporation - All rights reserved.

This document is geared towards providing helpful and reliable information in regards to the topic and issue covered. The publication is sold with the idea that the publisher is not required to render accounting, officially permitted, or otherwise, qualified services. If advice is necessary, legal or professional, a practiced individual in the profession should be ordered.

- From a Declaration of Principles which was accepted and approved equally by a Committee of the American Bar Association and a Committee of Publishers and Associations.

In no way is it legal to reproduce, duplicate, or transmit any part of this document in either electronic means or in printed format. Recording of this publication is strictly prohibited and any storage of this document is not allowed unless with written permission from the publisher. All rights reserved.

The information provided herein is stated to be truthful and consistent, in that any liability, in terms of inattention or otherwise, by any usage or abuse of any policies, processes, or directions contained within is the solitary and utter responsibility of the recipient reader. Under no circumstances will any legal responsibility or blame be held against the publisher for any reparation, damages, or monetary loss due to the information herein, either directly or indirectly.

Respective authors own all copyrights not held by the publisher.

The information herein is offered for informational purposes solely, and is universal as so. The presentation of the information is without contract or any type of guarantee assurance.

The trademarks that are used are without any consent, and the publication of the trademark is without permission or backing by the trademark owner. All trademarks and brands within this book are for clarifying purposes only and are the owned by the owners themselves, not affiliated with this document.

Table Of Contents

Introduction

I want to thank you and congratulate you for purchasing the book, *"Paleo Free Guide for Beginners: Over 50 Paleo Free Recipes for Optimal Health & Fast Weight Loss"*.

This book contains everything you might need to know when it comes to getting started with the Paleo Free Diet. It is provided in an easily digestible format that allows you to better absorb the information. There are no complicated explanations about how it works! You'll be given what you need straight up so you won't have to waste time trying to understand exactly what the diet is. Whether it's for your overall good health or to lose a few pounds, Paleo can certainly help you with it. To help you get started, we'll do the same and start you off with 50 of the best Paleo recipes that you can slowly but surely shift your everyday menu to.

It's never easy changing a diet. I often fall into self-pity when I can no longer have the foods I enjoy. Either I feel sorry for myself or I get rebellious and binge and anything and everything. I always knew the value of eating healthy. I could just never bring myself to do it. It wasn't until I had a miscarriage that I got serious about my health. I have made drastic changes that others just don't understand. But the payoff is the weight I've lost and the better health I'm experiencing.

My hope for you is not to be on another "diet." This isn't a restriction diet like Atkins. The goal is to have a lifestyle change. Lifestyle changes are more sustainable and maintain weight loss long term compared to restriction diets. The change is hard to start but worth it when you commit. The trick is to get the momentum to start.

Thanks again for purchasing this book. I hope you enjoy reading it and eating the recipes from it! Please take some time to stop by and LIKE our Facebook page:

https://www.facebook.com/joypublishing

With gratitude,

Emma Rose

Chapter 1 – What Is the Paleo Free Diet?

The Paleo Free Diet is known by many names such as the cavemen diet, stone age diet and hunter-gatherer diet, to name a few. The concept behind this diet follows that of the Paleolithic era before the development of agriculture. Essentially, you consume the same foods that the cavemen used to eat. The focus is on eating food closest to its natural, unprocessed state. The cavemen would gather their food from any source available whether it was wild animals, berries, vegetables, or fruits. As a result, they were strong, fit, and healthy for thousands of years.

This type of diet is still very young, less than fifty years only, but more in depth researches and studies are being conducted to increase the information and knowledge on this diet. The results of previous studies conducted on the Paleo Free Diet reveal the improvement of health to the people involved. This is attributed to the fact that no processed foods and additives are included. The Paleo Free Diet is a diet that works with our genetics – before machinery and processing got involved. Foods that were not available during the Paleolithic time such as dairy products, salt, sugar and grains are not included in the preparation of the Paleo Free Diet.

The modern diet predominately consumed in the Western world is full of refined foods, trans fats, salt and sugar. These ingredients are known to indirectly cause diseases such as hypertension, diabetes, strokes, obesity and other heart problems. The list goes on even further with the increase diagnosis of cancer, Parkinson's, Alzheimer's, depression and infertility. "What an extraordinary achievement for a civilization: to have developed the one diet that reliably makes its people sick!" (Michael Pollen, Food Rules: An Eater's Manual, Penguin Books 2009).

Foods included in the Paleo Free Diet

- Fruit

- Vegetables

- Lean Meat

- Seafood

- Nuts/Seeds

- Healthy Fats (eg. coconut, avocado, nuts and seeds, olive oil, grass fed butter)

Foods NOT included in the Paleo Free Diet

- Dairy

- Grain

- Processed Food

- Processed and Artificial Sugar

- Legumes (all beans, peas, peanuts, miso, lentils, soybeans, tofu)

- Starches (potatoes, sweet potatoes, yucca, butternut squash, acorn squash, yam, beets)

- Alcohol

- Soft Drinks

- Fruit Juices (high in sugar)

- Fatty Meats (eg. spam and hot dogs)

- Too Salty (eg. French fries and ketchup)

Why not grain?

You may be surprised to see that grains are not included in the Paleo Free Diet. We are accustomed to grains being a part of a balanced diet. However, our bodies are not designed to deal with the nutritional components of grains such as gluten, lectin, and phytates.

Gluten is a protein substance found in wheat, barley and rye. Many people are discovering that their bodies are gluten sensitive and are eliminating gluten from their diet. The most extreme case of gluten sensitivity is Celiac Disease. Individuals with this disease can pick up the minutest trace of gluten and react immediately.

Lectin binds to insulin receptors and can also cause leptin resistance.

Phytates cause minerals to become unavailable during digestion.

Why is dairy a problem?

When purchasing milk, you need to be mindful of the source. Milk from cows that are fed a grain diet is toxic. Animals are healthiest on a grass diet. However, when cattle consume a diet high in grains, they become inflamed, sick, fat and toxic, which then passes through to the milk. Due to the "toxicity" in the milk, it goes through a pasteurization process in order to kill the bad bacteria. Consequently, the good bacteria get killed as well. The result is dead processed milk that creates digestive problems for the milk drinker. It is best to drink raw unpasteurized milk in moderation. If you opt for not drinking milk, make sure to get your calcium from leafy green vegetables such as kale, broccoli and spinach.

Chapter 2 – Benefits of the Paleo Free Diet

"My health is the main capital I have and I want to administer it intelligently" – Earnest Hemingway

The Paleo Free Diet has massively gained in popularity because of its fantastic benefits due to sticking to the basic diet our ancestors consumed – a diet our bodies were built to handle.

Your body will benefit in the following ways when you follow the Paleo Free Diet:

- Normalized blood sugar levels

- Fat reduction

- More efficient workouts

- Lessened allergies

- Sustained energy levels

- Smoother skin

- Healthier teeth

- Restful sleep

- Sharper mind

What to expect

You can expect to see weight loss in the first month. Be mindful that this is usually water weight that is being shed. As you continue on with the diet, the body will start to burn the unwanted fat that's been built up over time. Don't be surprised when you start to experience withdrawal symptoms. These symptoms can last up to 3 weeks. Symptoms include:

- Nausea

- Headaches

- Irritability/Mood Swings

- Fatigue

- Intense Cravings

- Diarrhea/Constipation

- Flu-like symptoms

- Brain Fog

- Dizziness

- Increased Urination

- Increased Appetite/Thirst

You are not alone if you experience any of these symptoms. I myself felt worse before I felt better. At the 3 week point, I noticed a turn around and the symptoms cleared up. I felt nausea, fatigue, intense cravings, headaches, flu-like symptoms, increased urination and irritability. It's easy to want to give up when you feel so terrible but push through! It's worth being on the other side. Besides, it takes 21 days to break a habit. Set your mind for at least 21 days, you'll be glad you did.

I would also encourage you to keep track of your weight and waist measurements before you start so you can be motivated as you progress along. A before picture is a great idea too.

Chapter 3 – Food Rules

"All things in moderation including moderation" – Oscar Wilde

I stumbled upon the Paleo Free Diet because of my health journey with the naturopath. I was frustrated with my constant struggle with depression and fatigue. To top it off, I had a recent miscarriage. After my assessment with the doctor, I was told to remove wheat, corn, oats and dairy from my diet. In addition, I had to follow a diet that was 70% alkaline and 30% acidic. I left the doctor's office wondering, "What the heck can I eat?" I soon discovered that the Paleo Free Diet was the closest diet to the list of food restrictions I was trying to follow.

I started my diet choosing the food that I could and couldn't eat based on what the doctor said. I didn't completely get the heart behind why I was making these restrictive choices. Then my mind set began to shift and I started to embrace the "whys" behind why I was eating the way I was. I was beginning to become convicted of the benefits of eating in this manner.

Michael Pollan's book, *"Food Rules: An Eater's Manual,"* was introduced to me shortly after this journey began. I found many of his food rules to be realistic and refreshing. They contributed to this changing mind set that I was developing towards food. I wanted to share some of the food rules with you as well.

The overall conclusion of the book is the following 7 words:

"Eat food. Not too much. Mostly plants."

I like how he calls processed food "edible foodlike substances" because the name really calls the food for what it is: foodlike. This imagery helps me become turned off of all the junk food that I struggle to give up.

The rest of the book is broken down into 64 food rules based on what people should eat, the kind of food they should eat and how much they should eat. I created a list below of some of the food rules that I found eye opening.

• Don't eat anything your great-grandmother wouldn't recognize

• Avoid food products containing ingredients that no ordinary human would keep in the pantry

• Avoid high fructose corn syrup – this corn syrup is worse than sugar (sucrose)

• Do not eat food that has sugar within the top 3 ingredients

• Avoid food products that contain more than 5 ingredients

• Avoid food products that contain ingredients that are difficult to pronounce

• Avoid food products that make health claims (eg. reduces cholesterol or the chances of heart disease). These huge companies have money to do the research, vegetable farms do not. As a result, farmers are not able to boast about the health claims of their vegetables. You don't see a label on broccoli advertising its health claim. On the contrary, the absence of this label doesn't nullify its nutritional benefits.

• Eat foods cooked by humans and not corporations

12

- Don't ingest foods made in places where everyone is required to wear a surgical cap

- If it came from a plant, eat it; if its made in a plant, don't

- It's tot food if arrived from through the window of your car

- It's not food if it's called the same name in every language (eg. Big Mac)

- Eating what has no legs (fish) is better than eating what stands on one leg (plants) is better than eating what stands on 2 legs (poultry), which is better than eating what stands on 4 legs (cows, pigs, etc.)

- Avoid foods that are pretending to be something they are not (eg. margarine)

- Avoid foods advertised on TV

- Eat only foods that will eventually rot

- Eat food made from ingredients you can picture in its raw state or growing in nature

- Don't get your fuel from the same place your car does

- Spend as much time enjoying the meal as took to prepare

- Eat breakfast like a king, lunch like a prince, dinner like a pauper

- No snacks, no seconds, no sweets except on the days that begin with the letter "S"

- Break the rules once in a while or you'll go crazy

- Eat animals that have eaten well themselves

- Drink the spinach water – save the cooking water for soups and sauces

- Eat all the junk food you want as long as you cook it yourself

- Stop eating before your full – if you view your stomach like a bag, you need room to tie the bag closed. Eat until your 67-80% full.

- The banquet is in the first bite – it will never taste as good after that

- Eat sweet foods as you find them in nature

I expect some of these food rules triggered you in some way. My hope is for you to take them close to heart and incorporate them into your own life so you can eat as natural and wholesome as possible. Check out Michael Pollan's book, "Food Rules: An Eater's Manual" for more food rules

Chapter 4 – Paleo Smoothies and Beverages

Smoothies are great because they are quick to prepare and dense with nutrition. You can have a smoothie as a snack or meal replacement. There is a tonne of awesome add-ons you can use to make your smoothies that much more healthy.

Add-ons may include:

- 1 tablespoon maca

Maca is a super food that is native to the Andes Mountains. It is actually a root that is part of cruciferous family including broccoli, radish and water cress. 1 teaspoon of maca is only 10 calories! It has a nutty and earthy taste that complements smoothies. People use maca for enhancing fertility, boosting their immune system, stimulating their libido, or increasing energy.

- 1 tablespoon flax seed

Flax seeds are another super food that is considered one of the most powerful plant food on the plant. Flax seeds are high in fiber, omega-3 and lignans (reduces risk of breast or prostate cancer). Benefits of consuming flax seeds are a reduced risk of heart disease, diabetes, cancer, and stroke.

- 1 tablespoon chia seeds

Chia seeds are another super food that are a great source of protein, fiber and omega-3. The chia seeds are native to Mexico and Guatemala. They are the seeds that come from the flowering plant in the mint family. The health benefits of chia seeds include boosting energy, stabilizing blood sugar, reducing cholesterol, and assisting digestion.

- 1 serving of protein powder (not whey based)

- 1 serving of green super food powder such as spurlina

- Spices such as paprika, cinnamon, ginger or cayenne pepper

1. Raspberry Mojito Frappe

Ingredients:

- 1 ½ cup of frozen strawberries,

- 1 teaspoon of coconut or maple syrup,

- half a cup of orange juice,

- 6 pieces of mint leaves

How to:

Mix everything together using a blender. Add more or less liquid depending on the consistency you desire.

2. Toblerone Thickshake

Ingredients:

- 1/2 banana,
- 4 dried dates,
- 1/3 cup of hazelnuts,
- 1 tablespoon of cacao powder,
- 1 tablespoon of honey,
- 1 cup of almond or coconut milk,
- some ice cubes

How to:

Mix everything together using a blender. Add more or less liquid depending on the consistency you desire.

3. Tropical Avocado Smoothie

Ingredients:

- 1 avocado, peeled with pit removed,
- 1 cup of coconut cream,
- ½ a teaspoon of vanilla essence,
- 5 strawberries, hulled,
- 2/3 cup blueberries
- 1 banana, frozen
- 1/3 cup orange juice
- 1 cup of crushed or cubed ice

How to:

Process all of your ingredients in a blender and make sure it gets mixed well. Add more or less liquid depending on the consistency you desire.

4. Almost Pina Colada Drink

Ingredients:

- 1 cup pineapple juice,

- ½ a lime's juice,

- 1 cup of coconut milk,

- 1 banana

- a few cubes of ice

How to:

Process all of your ingredients in a blender until it gets mixed properly. Add more or less liquid depending on the consistency you desire.

5. Key Lime Pie Green Smoothie

Ingredients:

- 1 teaspoon of key lime zest,
- 2 tablespoon key lime juice,
- 1 ripe banana,
- 1 cup of unsweetened non-dairy milk,
- 2 drops of liquid Stevia,
- ¼ teaspoon of vanilla extract,
- 1 tablespoon sunflower butter,
- 2 cups of organic baby spinach,
- some ice cubes

How to:

Combine all of your ingredients in a blender and blend this for 30 seconds until it becomes smooth. Add more or less liquid depending on the consistency you desire. Optional topping: shredded coconut

6. Protein Smoothie

Ingredients:

- 4 small dates,

- 2 frozen bananas,

- 1 tablespoon of almond butter,

- 1/2 cup of hemp milk,

- 1 tablespoon of Chia seeds,

- ¼ cup water for thinning down the mix

How to:

Mix all of your ingredients in a blender and puree until it becomes smooth. Set this aside for some minutes so the Chia seeds can break down further (and provide you more nutrients) before serving. Add more or less liquid depending on the consistency you desire.

Chapter 5 – Paleo Breakfast

7. Homemade Paleo Granola

Ingredients:

- 1/3 cup of coconut oil,

- 1 ½ cups of coconut flour,

- 2 tsp nutmeg,

- 2 tsp cinnamon,

- ½ cup of coconut flakes,

- ½ cup of walnuts,

- ½ cup of hemp hearts,

- sea salt to taste

How to:

To start, preheat your over to 275°F. Combine all of your ingredients in a mixing bowl and thoroughly mix it together. A tip would be to melt the coconut oil first to make it easier to stir. Once done, spread this mixture this mixture in a single flat layer onto a greased baking sheet. Get rid of any air bubbles before baking it for about 40 minutes or 50 if you think it needs more toasting. Mix it every 10 minutes to make sure it is evenly baked. Once baked, allow it to cool before serving.

8. Primal Breakfast Burrito

Ingredients:

- 4 egg whites,

- 1 to 2 tomatoes depending on what you like, finely chopped,

- ½ an onion, finely chopped,

- 1 red pepper, cut into strips,

- ¼ cup of canned and diced green chilies,

- ½ a cup of cooked meat (you can use ground beef, sliced steak or shredded chicken),

- ¼ cup of chopped cilantro,

- hot sauce or some salsa on the side,

- 1 avocado cut into wedges

How to:

First, whisk your egg whites. Lightly oil a 10-inch skillet and warm this over low fire. Slowly pour half of your egg whites onto the pan, making sure to swirl it so that it gets spread evenly and thinly. Cook it for about a minute until it resembles a tortilla before removing it from the pan. This would be your burrito wrapper. Using the same pan, sauté your onions in oil before adding the red pepper, tomato, green chili and meat. Whisk more of the egg yolks into this and turn it into a scramble along with your other ingredients. Spoon half of this filling into your wrapper and roll it up nice, and tight. Add some avocados on top and serve with salsa or hot sauce.

9. Kale and Red Pepper Frittata

Ingredients:

- 1 tablespoon of coconut oil,

- half a cup of red pepper,

- 1/3 cup of onion,

- 2 cups of chopped and rinsed kale,

- 3 slices of chopped crispy bacon,

- 8 large eggs,

- half a cup of coconut or almond milk,

- salt and pepper to taste

How to:

To get started, preheat your over to 350°F and in a medium sized bowl, begin whisking your eggs and milk together. Add some salt and pepper according to your taste. Set this aside. Using a non-stick skillet, heat a tablespoon of the coconut over medium heat, to this add your red pepper and onion. Sauté it for 3 minutes or up until the onion becomes translucent. This when you'll add the kale, cooking it until the leaves wilt (this shouldn't take no more than 5 minutes). Lastly, add your eggs and bacon to the pan. Cook this mixture for 4 minutes or up until the edges and bottom of your frittata begins to set.

10.   Bacon Wrapped Eggs with Sweet Potato Hash

Ingredients:

- 4 eggs,

- 6 slices of bacon,

- 1 sweet potato,

- 1 tablespoon of olive oil,

- half a cup of onion,

- salt and pepper to taste

How to:

Preheat your oven to 375°F and in a small pan, sauté your bacon until it begins to brown but don't cook it fully. Take a muffin sheet and grease the bottoms of 4 slots, lining the edge of each one with a slice of bacon. Set the remaining 2 pieces aside since you'll need this for your sweet potato hash. Crack an egg into each of the 4 cups and bake it for at least 15 minutes. While you're waiting, make the hash by putting some olive oil, onions and sweet potato into a pan. Sauté this until the sweet potato softens. Lastly, chop up the remaining bacon and add it to the pan. Cook everything thoroughly then season with some salt and pepper.

11. Paleo Porridge

Ingredients:

- 2 whole eggs,

- 1 tablespoon of coconut flour,

- ½ cup of coconut milk (the creamier, the better),

- pinch of salt,

- seasoning (vanilla and cardamom would be good)

How to:

Put all of your ingredients together in a small pot and mix this well. Cook the mixture in the pot over low heat, continuously stirring until you get your desired texture.

12. Avocado Bacon Omelet

Ingredients:

- 4 bacon slices,

- 2 tablespoon red onion,

- 1 avocado,

- 1 tablespoon fresh cilantro,

- 4 eggs,

- 1 dash of hot sauce

How to:

Cook your bacon until it becomes crispy and while it's cooking, go and prepare your avocado. Half it and remove the pit, scooping the flesh into a bowl. Mash this until you get a nice texture. Add your cilantro and onion to it and once your bacon is done, drain and crumble the pieces into the avocado. Mix it all before making your omelets. Once done, put half of the avocado mixture on top and serve with hot sauce.

13. Vanilla and Orange Granola

Ingredients:

- 1 cup of raw pumpkin seeds,
- 2 cups of raw almonds,
- 1 cup coconut flakes,
- 1 cup raw sunflower seeds,
- ¼ cup of chia seeds,
- 1 tablespoon of ground vanilla,
- ½ cup of pure maple syrup,
- 1 tablespoon of orange zest,
- ¼ cup oil (olive, preferably),
- 1 cup of chopped dried apricots,
- ¼ cup apple butter

How to:

Preheat your oven to 275°F, add your almonds half a cup at a time to a food processor and pulse until it gets broken up. Transfer this along with the other ingredients except the apricot into a large bowl. Stir and make sure everything is evenly combined. Divide the granola evenly onto two baking sheets and bake for at least half an hour, stir at least 3 times, until it becomes golden brown. Remove and pour back into the bowl with the apricots. Allow to cool before serving.

14. Lemon Poppy seed Pancakes

Ingredients:

- 1/2 cup of coconut flour,

- 6 eggs,

- ¼ cup of maple syrup,

- ¼ cup of lemon juice,

- ¼ cup of coconut oil,

- 1 tablespoon of poppy seeds,

- the zest of two lemons,

- 1/2 teaspoon of baking soda,

- 2 tablespoons arrowroot starch,

- 1 teaspoon of cream of tartar

How to:

Using a large bowl, mix your coconut flour, eggs, coconut oil, maple syrup and your lemon juice. Stir well and then add your cream of tartar, poppy seeds and baking soda. Once you get a nice consistency, just take 2 spoonfuls of the mixture and start cooking your pancakes.

15. Dairy-Free Cream Cheese

Ingredients:

- 1 cup unsalted raw cashews, soaked

- 1 tablespoon lemon juice

- Dash of salt

- 1 teaspoon maple syrup (optional)

How to:

Soak unsalted raw cashews for a minimum of 6 hours. Overnight would be best. In a food processor, grind cashews until smooth with lemon juice and salt. Chill overnight. Experiment with the taste by adding maple syrup or another sweetener. Eat chilled.

16.Avocado and Strawberry Toast

Ingredients:

- 4 slices of bread (grain free),

- 2 ounces of dairy-free cream cheese,

- 1 avocado,

- a teaspoon of fresh lemon juice,

- 4 organic strawberries,

- a dash of salt

How to:

Start by toasting your bread. After, mash your avocado and add both lemon juice and salt to it. If you're using it, stir in your cream cheese. Mix this well before spreading it over your toast. Top this with slices of strawberry.

17. Cauliflower Breakfast Casserole

Ingredients:

- 10 organic eggs,

- 1 large cauliflower,

- 1 cup of organic or almond milk,

- Pinch of pepper,

- 1/2 teaspoon of salt,

- ¼ teaspoon of dried dill,

- 1 garlic

How to:

Steam your cauliflower until it softens. Combine your milk and eggs to it and whisk until it combines well. To this, add your salt, dill, pepper and garlic. Continue to stir. Drizzle a 13" x 9" baking dish with olive oil and put your steamed cauliflower on it. Pour the egg mixture onto it. Bake this at 350°F for 35 minutes or until it reaches the desired firmness.

Chapter 6 – Paleo Appetizers

18. Tomato Pesto Bites

Ingredients:

- Extra virgin olive oil,

- 30 cherry tomatoes,

- ¼ cup of toasted pine nuts,

- salt and pepper,

- 1 clove of garlic,

- 1 cup of some fresh basil

How to:

Wash and dry your tomatoes then slice a section of it its bottom, creating a flat surface so it can stand. Slice off the top and scoop out the seeds, keep the shape intact. Place all of your pesto ingredients in a food processor and mix this until smooth. Fill your tomatoes with pesto and drizzle with some olive oil, and a sprinkling of salt before serving.

19. Veggies with Spinach Artichoke Dip

Ingredients:

- 10 ounces frozen and chopped spinach,

- 2 x 14 ounce cans of artichoke hearts,

- half a red bell pepper,

- 1 teaspoon of garlic powder,

- 1/2 cup of cashew butter,

- 1 tablespoon of green onion,

- ¼ teaspoon of cayenne

- 1 teaspoon of salt

How to:

Cook your frozen spinach over medium heat, slowly breaking it up while it cooks. Add your red bell and artichokes, continuously cooking until everything is heated through. Then, mix your butter, cashew, garlic, cayenne, salt and green onion. Add this to your pan and stir thoroughly and evenly. Serve this with your choice of veggies or veggie chips.

20.   Spiced Kale Chips

Ingredients:

*   6 cups torn and stemmed kale ,

*   1 teaspoon of gingerbread spice mix or a pinch of paprika,

*   2 teaspoons olive oil or virgin coconut oil

*   salt for seasoning

How to:

Preheat your oven 350°F. Prepare your kale by removing stems and tearing up leaves into chip size pieces. Set aside. In another bowl, mix your gingerbread spice mix and olive oil. Pour this oil mix over your kale and mix well. Arrange your chips on a baking try lined with parchment paper. Bake for 12 to 15 minutes or until they get crispy. Let cool before serving.

21. Paleo Bacon Dip

Ingredients:

- 3 slices of bacon,

- 1 can of artichoke hearts,

- a handful of baby spinach,

- 1 ½ tablespoons of olive oil,

- 1/2 cup of cashews,

- 1/2 tablespoon of artichoke juice,

- 1/2 teaspoon of onion powder,

- ¼ teaspoon of dry mustard,

- ½ teaspoon of garlic powder ,

- ¼ teaspoon dry mustard

How to:

Crisp your bacon over medium heat then set it aside. Cut your artichokes lengthwise and sauté it with your spinach. Let this cool. Using a blender, powder your cashews the drizzle with olive oil. Add your seasoning and artichoke-spinach mix. Pulse a few times before stirring in your remaining ingredients. Serve this with homemade potato chips or vegetables.

22.   Rosemary Fried Almonds

Ingredients:

- 2 cups of blanched raw almonds,

- 2 teaspoons of salt,

- 2 tablespoons of minced fresh rosemary

- some coconut oil (or ghee)

How to:

To a large pan set over medium heat, pour some coconut oil and coat it evenly. Add your almonds and stir so they don't burn. Turn the heat down when the almonds turn golden brown and add your salt, and rosemary. Stir and cook until the rosemary becomes fragrant. Once done, drain the oil and serve.

23. Cajun Carrot Fries

Ingredients:

- 10 large carrots sliced like fries,

- ¼ teaspoon of cayenne powder,

- 1 tablespoon of olive oil,

- salt and pepper to season with

How to:

Preheat oven to 450°F then grease or your baking sheet. Toss your carrots with the cayenne pepper, salt, black pepper and olive oil. Arrange your fries on the sheet and bake this for 15 minutes, then flip over and repeat the baking process. Serve warm.

24.   Spicy Parsnip Wedges

Ingredients:

- 3 wedged parsnips,

- ½ teaspoon of black pepper,

- ½ teaspoon of salt,

- ½ teaspoon of cumin,

- 3 tablespoons of coconut oil,

- 1 teaspoon of paprika,

- 1 garlic, minced,

- ¼ teaspoon of cayenne powder

How to:

Place your wedges in a bowl and pour coconut oil over this, stir and coat well. Sprinkle the rest of your ingredients over it and stir once more. Transfer this to a line cookie sheet or tray and bake at 400°F for half an hour, or until it becomes soft and golden.

25.   Baked Jicama Fries

Ingredients:

- 1 jicama (Mexican yam or turnip),

- 1 teaspoon of salt,

- 1 tablespoon of olive oil,

- 1 teaspoon of black pepper,

- 1 teaspoon of red pepper,

- 1 teaspoon of salt

How to:

Preheat your oven to 450°F and cut your jicama in half. Slice the stem and cast aside. Chop your jicama into lengthwise fries. Set this on a baking sheet, splash some olive oil over it and sprinkle your remaining ingredients all over it evenly. Bake for 15 minutes or until golden.

Chapter 7 – Paleo Soups

26.   **Paleo Chicken Tortilla Soup**

Ingredients:

- 2 large chicken breasts with the skin removed, cut into half inch strips,

- 32 ounces of organic chicken broth,

- 28oz can of tomatoes, diced,

- 1 sweet onion, diced,

- a bunch of cilantro, finely chopped,

- 2 tablespoons of tomato paste,

- 4 cloves of garlic, minced,

- 1 teaspoon of cumin,

- 1 teaspoon of chili powder,

- olive oil,

- fresh pepper and sea salt,

- 1 (or 2, depending on the need) cups of water

How to:

In a large Dutch oven (or a Crockpot) over medium high heat, add a dash of your favorite olive oil as well as ¼ cup of chicken broth. To this, you will also need to add your onions, jalapenos, garlic, pepper and sea salt. Cook these until it becomes soft and add more broth as you see fit. Once that's done, you have to add all the remaining ingredients and just enough water to fill the container. Cover this and allow it to cook on low heat for about 2 hours, tasting and adding seasoning whenever needed. After your chicken has been fully cooked, shredding it should be easier. Top this with some avocado slices and cilantro before serving.

27.   Hunter Stew

Ingredients:

- 2 pounds of cubed beef,

- a handful of fresh berries (you can add more as you see fit),

- 2 baby carrots, sliced,

- coconut oil,

- butter,

- 1 onion, sliced,

- salt, pepper,

- garlic powder,

- oregano,

- red wine or Worcestershire sauce (optional)

How to:

Brown your beef in the coconut oil and put it on a medium simmer along with your onions, allowing it to slowly soften up. Once done, add your seasoning and add more as you see fit. You can also toss in the carrots and if you want to, half a cup of the red wine along with a splash of your Worcestershire sauce. Make sure that you add enough water so your meat is covered. Let this stew for about 30 minutes. You can add your berries at the last minute as well as a teaspoon of butter to coat it. Once your carrots are tender, serve the dish.

28.   Roasted Tomato Soup

Ingredients:

- 4 ripe tomatoes,

- half a yellow onion,

- 1 tablespoon of olive oil,

- 5 garlic cloves,

- 1 tablespoon of chopped parsley,

- 2 tablespoon of tomato paste,

- 1 ½ cups of vegetable broth,

- salt and pepper for seasoning

How to:

Begin by preheating your oven to 350°F. After, cut your onion and tomatoes into wedges then spread these on a baking sheet. Over it, drizzle some olive oil before sprinkling your seasoning and chopped parsley. Toss it together with your hands before tucking the cloves into a tomato so they don't burn. Roast this for about 40 minutes then let cool. Warm the broth over medium heat before stirring in some of the tomato paste. Add the roasted ingredients and let simmer for 8 minutes. After this, transfer to a food processor and blend until it becomes smooth. Add salt and pepper as you see fit.

29.   Chicken Avocado Soup

Ingredients:

- 6 cups of chicken broth,

- 1 pound of boneless and skinless chicken breast,

- 4 scallions,

- 1 teaspoon hot sauce,

- 1 diced avocado,

- 1 garlic clove,

- salt and black pepper for seasoning

How to:

Pour your broth into a saucepan and place this over medium heat. Add your hot sauce and stir. While the broth cooks, dice your chicken and slice your scallions. Stir this into the broth along with the garlic. Bring it back to a simmer and leave for 10 minutes. Add your seasoning before serving.

Chapter 8 – Paleo Meals

30.   Paleo Sausage Balls

Ingredients:

- A pound of sausage (you can use homemade ones too),

- 2 large eggs,

- ¼ cup of coconut flour,

- 1 teaspoon of baking soda

How to:

Preheat your oven to 350°F while you combine all of the ingredients. A mixer with a simple paddle attachment would make your work more efficient. Once mixed thoroughly, you can then form this into balls about 1 ¼ inches when it comes to diameter. Place these on a greased baking sheet then bake them for at least 20 minutes.

31. Stegosaurus Sandwich

Ingredients:

- 1 large purple sweet potato,

- ¼ teaspoon of paprika,

- 3 tablespoons of olive oil, 4 if you prefer,

- ¼ teaspoon of cumin,

- half a teaspoon of garlic powder,

- salt for seasoning

How to:

Preheat your oven to 450°F and place a steel drying rack over a cookie sheet. Using a small bowl, combine all of your spices. In a larger one, toss your potato slices together with the olive oil so it gets coated. Once done, sprinkle your spice mixture over the potatoes and stir it so it gets evenly coated. Bake this for about half an hour to 40 minutes until it gets crispy. Sprinkle with more salt if you want to before removing it from the oven. Let it cool for a bit before serving.

32.   Easy Paleo Chicken Stir-fry

Ingredients:

2 cooked and shredded chicken breasts,

2 sliced bell peppers,

¼ teaspoon of chili powder,

1 tablespoon of coconut aminos (coconut sap) or substitute soy sauce,

1 tablespoon of coconut oil

Salt and pepper for seasoning

How to:

On a frying pan over medium heat, add a tablespoon of coconut oil and soften your bell peppers in it. Once soft enough, add your cooked chicken meat before adding the coconut aminos (or soy sauce), salt, pepper and chili powder. Simply mix it all together, and stir-fry for at least five more minutes.

33.   Sesame Seed Crusted Snapper

Ingredients:

- 6 to 7 ounces Red snapper, filleted and skinned,

- 1 tablespoon of sesame seeds,

- kosher or sea salt,

- fresh black pepper (cracked),

- 1 tablespoon of grass-fed butter or bacon fat

How to:

Dust one side of the snapper fillet with a mixture of kosher salt and pepper before laying this on top of the sesame seeds. Press down to ensure an even coating. Do the same to the other side. In a frying pan, melt a teaspoon of the butter. Increase the heat before putting the snapper in the pan, cooking each side for at least 3 to 4 minutes. The seeds should take on a golden color.

34.   Japanese Style Hamburger

Ingredients:

- A pound of organic grass fed ground beef,

- 3 cloves of garlic,

- 1 shallot,

- 1 egg,

- ¼ white onion, diced,

- white and black pepper,

- coconut aminos (coconut sap),

- salt

How to:

Using a food processor or a mortar and pestle, ground your shallot, garlic and onion. Mix this together with your ground beef; add your eggs and all of your seasoning after. Heat your skillet using medium heat, divide your mixture into 4 patties and pan sear it until it's brown. Flip it every now and then but do not squeeze so it retains the juices. Add about a tablespoon of water before adding the coconut aminos. Allow this to simmer for 2 minutes. Turn the heat up to reduce the sauce and once done, serve.

35. Meat Crust Pizza

Ingredients ("Crust"):

• 2 pounds of Italian sausage (or any other of your preference)

• 1 to 2 whole eggs

Ingredients (Topping):

• Sugarless pizza sauce,

• Onions, chopped,

• bell peppers, chopped,

• broccoli, chopped,

• garlic, chopped,

• mushrooms, chopped,

• zucchini, chopped,

• olives, chopped,

• You'll also need cheese, try making almond cheese

How to:

Heat your oven to 375°F while you mix the eggs and sausage. It would be best to use your hands for this. Once done, pat this into an iron skillet or a baking dish that's been lightly oiled. Set it into the fire for at least 25 minutes. This would be your crust. After it cooks, bring it out and top it with the pizza sauce, sprinkle the veggies and cheese over it. Some oregano would be good too before popping it back to the over for another 10 to 15 minutes. Let it cool before serving.

36.   Honey Orange Chicken

Ingredients:

- 1 pound chicken breast, cubed,

- 2 tablespoons of garlic,

- 2 tablespoons of ginger,

- 2 tablespoons of honey,

- 2 tablespoons of coconut aminos,

- 1 tablespoon of chili sauce,

- half a cup of orange juice,

- green onions, chopped,

- fish sauce for seasoning

How to:

Stir fry your chicken in the coconut oil until it begins to brown. Add your garlic and ginger then sauté for 1 minute. Lower your heat and add the liquid ingredients. Stir everything to coat the chicken evenly and allow to simmer until the sauce thickens. Serve with green onions.

37.   Japanese Beef and Bamboo

Ingredients:

- Minced beef,

- a jar of bamboo shoots,

- spinach,

- garlic,

- green beans,

- ginger,

- fish sauce,

- black pepper,

- chili,

- coconut oil

How to:

Cook your beef depending on how you like your meat. If you want it well-cooked, brown your beef in a lidded pan with a dash of coconut oil to the mix as well as a pint of water if it seems too dry. Close the lid and lower the heat, allowing it to cook for an hour (or longer). Drain the bamboo shoots while the beef was still cooking. To your beef, add the ginger, chili, garlic, fish sauce, black pepper and green beans. Stir this and place the lid back. Once you notice a reduction in the liquid, add your spinach and wait for it to wilt, as well as for the liquid to reduce completely.

38.   Turkish Menemen

Ingredients:

- 1 medium tomato,

- ¼ diced onion,

- ½ a cup of green bell pepper,

- 1 garlic clove,

- 1 tablespoon of olive oil,

- ¼ teaspoon of the following: cumin, turmeric, black pepper, red pepper flakes and salt,

- 3 eggs,

- 1 tablespoon of fresh parsley

How to:

Sauté your tomato, onion and parsley over low heat using olive oil. Crush your garlic and add it in along with the spices. Stir it often to mix well and keep until the vegetables begin to soften. While this is cooking, prepare your eggs by whisking them in a separate bowl. Once done, pour this in with your vegetables and scramble. This should be creamy. Cook until it softly sets and transfer to a plate. Top with parsley.

39.   Ceviche

Ingredients:

- 2 pounds of cubed fish fillets,

- 8 garlic cloves,

- 10 limes,

- 1 habanero chili,

- 1 tablespoon fresh cilantro,

- 1 red onion,

- 16 large lettuce leaves,

- 2 tomatoes,

- 2 avocados,

- salt and black pepper,

- hot sauce

How to:

Juice your limes using a food processor making sure to avoid the membrane. Add your cilantro and garlic. Seed your hot pepper and remove the white ribs before adding this to your food processor. Pulse these until both pepper and garlic are finely minced and pour this over your fish. Slice your onions and add it to the fish as well. Let this marinate in the fridge overnight before cooking. Be sure to add salt and pepper before you serve.

40.   Asian Pepper Shrimp

Ingredients:

- 4 cloves of garlic, minced,

- 3 tablespoons of coconut,

- 1 ½ pound of peeled shrimp,

- 1 tablespoon fish sauce,

- 1 tablespoon coconut aminos (coconut sap),

- 1 teaspoon of black pepper

- ¼ cup of fresh cilantro

How to:

Melt your coconut oil over low heat and add your garlic to this. Stir it for 2 minutes and keep your heat low. Add your shrimp and sauté until it turns pink then add your fish sauce, coconut aminos and pepper. Sauté this some more before transferring to a plate. Pour the liquid and oil over your shrimp and top with cilantro before serving.

41. Crunchy Deviled Chicken

Ingredients:

- ½ a cup of almond meal,

- 4 chicken legs,

- 1 teaspoon cayenne,

- 1 teaspoon of curry powder,

- 1 teaspoon dry mustard,

- 4 tablespoon of olive oil

How to:

Preheat your oven to 350°F. On a plate, combine your seasonings with the almond meal. Rub each chicken piece with some olive oil and let it roll over your almond meal and seasoning. Evenly arrange it on your roasting pan and roast it for an hour or up until the juices turn clear. The coating should be crunchy.

42.   Asparagus and Bacon

Ingredients:

- 1 pound of bacon,

- a bunch of asparagus,

- lemon juice,

- salt and pepper

How to:

Start by slicing your bacon, ¼ inch for each piece. Brown these in a pan over medium heat and set aside once you content with the way they've cooked. Keep about 2 tablespoons of the grease from the pan: you'll use the grease for sautéing the asparagus. Cut your greens to 1 inch pieces and discard the first couple of inches at the end of the stalks. Toss them in the same pan as the bacon and sauté for no more than 15 minutes. Add your bacon into the mix, season with some salt and pepper then serve.

43. Spinach and Ham Omelet with Spicy Piperade

Ingredients (Omelet):

- Coconut oil,

- 2 eggs already beaten,

- salt and pepper,

- 1 cup ham, cubed,

- at least a handful of baby spinach torn into small pieces

How to (Omelet):

Melt your coconut oil using a small sauté pan then add your eggs. Season this with some salt and pepper. Cook it until your egg has set then sprinkle it with ham and pile on the spinach to one side, folding until you're done. Top this with piperade.

Ingredient (Piperade):

3 cloves of garlic,

a large onion,

3 tablespoons of olive oil,

4 sprigs of thyme,

1 red bell pepper,

1 yellow bell pepper,

1 red chilli,

1 cup of cherry tomatoes,

1 teaspoon of salt

How to (Piperade):

Sauté your garlic, onions and thyme in the olive oil and wait until your onion begins to soften. After, add your chilli and peppers, continue to sauté this for at least 3 more minutes before finally adding the tomatoes. Sprinkle some salt to taste before covering and letting it simmer for at least 5 minutes.

Chapter 9 – Paleo Salads

44.   Balsamic Green Bean Salad

Ingredients:

- 1 ½ pounds of green beans, trimmed and cut,

- 3 tablespoons of olive oil,

- half a red onion, chopped,

- 2 tablespoons of balsamic vinegar,

- 1/3 cup of chopped walnuts,

- salt and pepper for seasoning

How to:

Boil a pot of salted water and add the green beans to it, blanching it for about 2 to 3 minutes. These should be barely cooked through and still have that crispiness. After, prepare a bowl of ice water and transfer the beans to this bowl. Drain after. Once done, simply place your red onion and green beans into another bowl, tossing it in olive oil. Sprinkle some balsamic into it and season with some pepper and salt. Top everything with walnuts before serving.

45.   Mango Avocado Spiced Chicken Salad

Ingredients:

- 1 small lettuce,

- 1 to 2 cups of shredded chicken,

- 1 diced avocado,

- 1 diced mango,

- ½ a teaspoon of cumin,

- ½ a teaspoon of chili powder,

- salt and pepper for seasoning

How to:

Place your lettuce in a bowl and do the same to your chicken in a separate one. Add a tiny bit of water to your chicken to keep it moist before microwaving for at least 15 seconds. Add the chili and cumin to this and mix. Once done, add it to your lettuce and simply top with some avocados, and mangoes. You can add a light dressing such as olive oil and lemon juice, or eat as is.

46.   Twisted Apple Coleslaw

Ingredients:

- ¼ head of green cabbage,

- ¼ head of red cabbage,

- 3 stalks of green onion,

- 2 diced honey crisp apples,

- half an avocado,

- a handful of walnuts,

- half a lemon (juiced),

- ¼ cup of apple cider vinegar,

- ¼ cup of walnut oil,

- salt and pepper for seasoning

How to:

Mash up your avocado and mix it with the lemon, oil, salt, pepper and vinegar. Chop up the other ingredients and transfer these to a bowl. Add the avocado "dressing" and place it in the fridge for half an hour. Adjust your seasoning if needed.

47.   Tuna Salad

Ingredients:

- 1 avocado,

- the juice of 1 lemon,

- 5 ounce of drained tuna,

- 1 tablespoon celery,

- 1 tablespoon chopped onion,

- 1 tablespoon of parsley,

- 1 tablespoon of shredded carrot,

- 4 cups of organic mix greens,

- salt and pepper for seasoning

How to:

Mash your avocado and combines this with your lemon juice, add the rest of your ingredients to this carefully after. Add salt and pepper according to your taste. Place your greens on a plate and spoon your tuna mix on top.

48.   Detox Salad

Ingredients:

- 4 cups of shredded kale,

- 4 cups of shredded cabbage,

- ½ a cup of fresh cilantro,

- 2 cups of shredded carrots,

- juice of 2 lemons,

- ½ a cup of raw almond butter,

- 2 teaspoon fresh grated ginger,

- ¼ cup of apple cider vinegar

How to:

In a big salad bowl, toss your kale, cabbage, cilantro and carrots together. Set this aside and whisk the vinegar, butter, ginger and lemon juice together. Pour this dressing over your salad and toss again.

49.   Simple Mushroom Salad

Ingredients:

- 2 marinated cucumbers,

- 350 grams of marinated mushrooms,

- 1 middle-sized onion,

- 1 boiled potato,

- Pinch of salt,

- 2 tablespoons sunflower seed oil

How to:

Drain your mushrooms, chopping them after. Cut your onions into half rings, dice both cucumbers and potato. Mix all of your ingredients together; add your oil and salt. Serve.

50.   Fruity Cabbage Salad

Ingredients:

- ½ a head of grated cabbage,

- 1 diced apple,

- 1 carrot,

- 1/3 cup chopped parsley

For your dressing:

- 1 pitted and peeled orange,

- 1 tablespoon of apple cider vinegar,

- ½ a cup of coconut cream,

- ¼ teaspoon ginger powder,

- salt and pepper for seasoning

How to:

Combine all of your salad ingredients in one bowl. In a different one, mix all of your dressing ingredients and blend until it becomes smooth. Pour this over your salad, toss and serve.

Chapter 10 – Paleo Desserts (Bonus recipes from the book, "Paleo Desserts")

51.   Choco Cookies

Ingredients:
- 1 ½ cups almonds

- ¼ tsp baking soda

- ¼ tsp sea salt

- ½ cup chocolate chips

- 2 tbsp coconut oil

- ½ tsp vanilla

- ½ cup maple syrup

- 1 egg

How To:

In a bowl, combine the following ingredients: 1 ½ cups almond, ¼ teaspoon baking soda, ¼ teaspoon sea salt and ½ cup chocolate chips. In a separate bowl, mix the following: 2 tablespoon coconut oil, ½ teaspoon vanilla. ½ cup maple syrup, 1 egg. Combine the two mixtures and let the batter stay in the refrigerator for 30 minutes.

While waiting for the batter, line the baking sheet with parchment paper. The oven should be preheated to 350°F. Place the batter onto the sheet according to the size of the cookies that you like. Bake for 5 minutes. Take the baking sheet out of the oven and flatten each cookie. Put the baking sheet back for another 5 minutes. Let it cool before serving.

52. Blackberry Cobbler

Ingredients:

- 3 cups fresh blackberries

- Honey

- 1 ½ cups finely ground almonds

- 2 tbsp coconut oil

- Cinnamon, to taste

How To:

Place 3 cups of fresh blackberries in a pie pan. Drizzle a bit of honey on top of the berries. In a separate bowl, mix 1 ½ cups finely ground almonds and 2 tablespoon coconut oil plus add cinnamon according to your taste preference (maybe a pinch or a teaspoon). Mix well. You would expect the mixture to be thick and clumpy. Crumble this on top of the berries and bake for 35 minutes at 350°F.

Check out the rest of "Paleo Desserts: Satisfy Your Sweet Tooth With Over 100 Quick and Easy Paleo Dessert Recipes and Paleo Baking Recipes" on Amazon

Or go to: http://amzn.to/1lZNcVI

Conclusion

Thank you again for purchasing this book!

I hope this book was able to help you get started when it comes to losing weight through the Paleo Free Diet.

The next step is to try the recipes and incorporate them into your daily diet to get the ball rolling towards a healthier and fitter lifestyle.

I would love for you to share your experiences, stories and encouragements with me. My email address is emmarosekindle@gmail.com

Finally, if you enjoyed this book and found it meaningful, please take the time to share your thoughts and post a positive review on Amazon. I greatly appreciate your time and effort.

In addition, please remember to check out our Facebook page in order to find other resources and upcoming promotions:

https://www.facebook.com/joypublishing

With sincere thanks,

Emma Rose

Preview Of "Paleo Desserts: Satisfy Your Sweet Tooth With Over 100 Quick and Easy Paleo Dessert Recipes and Paleo Baking Recipes"

Introduction

I want to thank you for purchasing the book, "Paleo Desserts: Satisfy Your Sweet Tooth With Over 100 Quick and Easy Paleo Dessert Recipes and Paleo Baking Recipes".

This book contains 100 Paleo dessert and baking recipes on how to prepare delectable desserts without sacrificing your health.

All my life I've had a sweet tooth. I would even go as far as to say that I had a sugar addiction! Over the last few years my sugar addiction got worse: I had dessert multiple times a day and every day (I guess being a Foods teacher didn't help much). I would joke with people by telling them that I had my servings of vegetables for the day in chocolate...except, I still didn't have the vegetables. It got pretty bad. I knew I hated eating that much dessert but I couldn't stop. I would eat one Ferrero Rochers and then go back for another. As I walked back to the treats, I would pass the mirror and think to myself, "I don't need to have this chocolate. But, ah, what the heck, I don't care." In the end, I'd have about 6 Ferrero Rochers in addition to the other treats I had earlier that day.

Finally, I had to take the huge tray of Ferrero Rochers to school to give to my students on Valentine's Day. There was no way I could eat the other 30 myself. Eating all this sugar caused a huge war within me. I knew that my extreme sugar eating was unhealthy for me but I didn't want to stop. I loved it too much. As a result, I wrestled between the ideal of where I wanted to be and the reality of where I was. I knew I had the discipline to say no to other things, so why couldn't I say no to chocolate?

I eventually came to the point where I was starting to get fed up with not feeling well. I had a lot of chronic pain in my neck and I was constantly tired. I knew that sugar was irritating the problem and causing inflammation in my body. At was starting to reach the breaking point. Ultimately, I chose to go off of sugar for at least three weeks to break the habit I had created for myself. It was seriously a miracle to stay consistent with my goal because I really didn't want to give up my favorite desserts.

Shortly after my decision to go off of sugar, I had a miscarriage. Experiencing the loss catapulted me into a massive journey to find health and proper nutrition. I did a live blood analysis with a naturopath to discover what was contributing to the terrible ways I was feeling. Seeing all the garbage I had in my blood forced me to go off of dairy, corn, oats, and wheat. I was left wondering, "What the heck am I going to eat? That stuff is in everything!"

Consequently, I stumbled upon the Paleo Free Diet. It was the most relevant diet to what I was trying to accomplish. I was able to find things to eat for breakfast, lunch and dinner. But desserts were a whole other story. I felt like something was missing and I couldn't put my finger on it. The best I could come up with was apple slices dipped in almond butter: hardly satisfying. Paleo desserts ended up being the by-product of my search to find something, anything that I could enjoy.

I encourage you to make that switch to healthier and happier desserts with the hundred delicious and irresistible recipes presented in this book. You don't need to follow the same extremity that I did. But if you are taking the Paleo Free Diet seriously, then you may find the same void of sweets in your life too. Cutting out all the processed foods and going back to the basics really does clear up the body and help it function better. I've seen the changes in my own life as hard as it's been to make those changes. You, too, can make the changes necessary and still have your sweets along the way!

Thank you again for purchasing this book. I hope you enjoy the recipes. Experiment with them and make substitutions to suit your needs.

With gratitude,

Emma Rose

Chapter 1

Brief History of Paleo Free Diet

The Sweet Effects

Why do you love sweet food? Why do you crave for more of that dessert so much? Your anatomy would tell you that sweet foods would cause the release of dopamine in the part of the brain that is associated with motivation and reward. Not only that, but studies show that sweets also produce an increased level of serotonin. Serotonin gives you that feeling of happiness and wellbeing. That's why it is better to give a box of chocolates when you want the person to be in a good mood.

Unfortunately, the quote you can't have your cake and eat it too applies here. The bad effects that sugar brings are common knowledge. The number one disease is diabetes. People are aware of diabetes and its complications. That is why even when you intensely crave for that delicious dessert, you try to control your urges and settle for nothing instead. Well, that is if your self-control is in good condition. More often than not, people would rather risk the medical condition and eat that sweet thing with all their heart.

I have had many slip ups in my own life. I went two months without chocolate...can you believe it? Then Easter came. I found that if I gave myself an inch, I would take a mile. Eating chocolate quickly got out of control. I rebelled because I was strict for so long. You may find yourself in the same situation and find it hard

94

to balance the sugar cravings. Once the sugar cravings are there, your body craves more and then a vicious cycle begins.

Check out the rest of "Paleo Desserts: Satisfy Your Sweet Tooth With Over 100 Quick and Easy Paleo Dessert Recipes and Paleo Baking Recipes" on Amazon.

Or go to: http://amzn.to/1lZNcVI

Detox Diet Guide

Lose Weight Quickly, Achieve Optimal Health and Feel Energized Through the 10 Day Detox

Emma Rose

© Copyright 2014 by Joy Publishing & Marketing Corporation - All rights reserved.

This document is geared towards providing helpful and reliable information in regards to the topic and issue covered. The publication is sold with the idea that the publisher is not required to render accounting, officially permitted, or otherwise, qualified services. If advice is necessary, legal or professional, a practiced individual in the profession should be ordered.

- From a Declaration of Principles which was accepted and approved equally by a Committee of the American Bar Association and a Committee of Publishers and Associations.

In no way is it legal to reproduce, duplicate, or transmit any part of this document in either electronic means or in printed format. Recording of this publication is strictly prohibited and any storage of this document is not allowed unless with written permission from the publisher. All rights reserved.

The information provided herein is stated to be truthful and consistent, in that any liability, in terms of inattention or otherwise, by any usage or abuse of any policies, processes, or directions contained within is the solitary and utter responsibility of the recipient reader. Under no circumstances will any legal responsibility or blame be held against the publisher for any reparation, damages, or monetary loss due to the information herein, either directly or indirectly.

Respective authors own all copyrights not held by the publisher.

The information herein is offered for informational purposes solely, and is universal as so. The presentation of the information is without contract or any type of guarantee assurance.

The trademarks that are used are without any consent, and the publication of the trademark is without permission or backing by the trademark owner. All trademarks and brands within this book are for clarifying purposes only and are the owned by the owners themselves, not affiliated with this document.

Table of Contents

Introduction

I want to thank you and congratulate you for purchasing the book, *"Detox Diet Guide: Lose Weight Quickly, Achieve Optimal Health and Feel Energized Through the 10 Day Detox"*.

This book contains proven steps and strategies on how to not just simply flush out toxic substances from our bodies, but to also enhance the way our bodies naturally flush out those toxins.

It also contains other important information such as the most common toxins that are found in the environment that we unknowingly consume, the many ways our bodies naturally detoxify themselves, the things one must and must not do within the ten days of the detox diet, detoxification recipes that can be easily prepared, and some important reminders that must be taken before, during, and after the detox diet.

Thanks again for purchasing this book. I hope you enjoy it! Please take some time to stop by and LIKE our Facebook page:

https://www.facebook.com/joypublishing

With gratitude,

Emma Rose

Chapter 1: Toxins and the Body

As the human body does its usual processes, some things need to be expelled. These are usually waste products made as a result of filtering out substances not needed by the body. There is a reason for the so-called "calls of nature" – which are peeing and releasing excrement.

But sometimes, those unwanted substances can build up in the organs and the bodily systems that comprise them. If there are too much of those substances, they will cause all sorts of harm to the overall bodily functions that can lead to various ailments.

The Top 10 List of Most Common Toxins

Human civilization evolves as a result of the desire of the people to live more comfortably and conveniently. But in the process of that evolution, it has unknowingly unleashed a cavalcade of impurities that do not just pollute the environment, but also the human body. Despite the many efforts by several government agencies and private individuals to thwart the sources of those impurities, there are traces of those impurities that still linger around. Those traces remain in the air, in the soil, in several bodies of water – and eventually, in the foods that humanity consumes.

According to Dr. Joseph Mercola, a well-known personality in the US wellness movement and owner and founder of Mercola.com (one of the most-trusted health websites), the ten most common toxic substances that are still prevalent in the environment to this day are the following:

1. Polychlorinated biphenyls, or PCBs, were commonly dumped by factories into nearby bodies of water. Due to their toxicity, PCBs were banned decades ago. However, traces of PCBs can still be found in those bodies of water since the toxic substances do not break down easily even after all those years. Fish that swim in those bodies of water still consume PCBs

unknowingly. As people still eat those fish, they will also ingest PCBs that will contribute to ailments such as cancer and brain defects in newborn babies.

2. Pesticides, while they do kill pests as their name says, are the major contributors of cancer. As farms still use synthetic pesticides such as weed killers, fungi killers, and insect killers; residues of those pesticides still remain in as much as 50 to 90 percent of US farm produce. Furthermore, there are bug sprays used to kill cockroaches and other unwanted insects in homes. Those bug sprays also contain the same carcinogenic substances as farm-focused pesticides. Besides cancer, pesticides also cause Parkinson's disease, miscarriage, nerve damage, birth defects, and getting in the way of nutrient absorption.

3. Fungal toxins not just come in the form of poisonous mushrooms. The most common of those fungal toxins is mold. Mold thrives in moist places such as bathrooms and kitchens; and can even sustain in vulnerable foods such as peanuts, wheat, and corn. One in three people are allergic to this fungal toxin. If left unchecked, mold causes cancer, heart disease, asthma, multiple sclerosis, and diabetes.

4. Phthalates are commonly found in plastic products and are responsible for softening them, making them easier to mold. They can seep into foodstuffs and drinks that are placed inside plastic food containers and plastic bottles. The result of ingesting too much phthalates is hormonal imbalance, since the substances resemble naturally-produced hormones. In children, phthalates can stunt their growth.

5. Volatile organic compounds, or VOCs, are commonly found in several household products such as air fresheners, cleaning fluids, mothballs, and varnishes. VOCs aid in air pollution and cause several sicknesses such as cancer, irritation of eyes and lungs, headaches, dizziness, and impaired memory.

6. Dioxins are some of the pollutants that are produced when something is burned, especially in massive quantities. As they

are released into the air, humans not just breathe in the dioxins. Livestock can also inhale those toxins and settle in their fats even after they are brought to the slaughterhouse to be made into meat. Dioxins cause cancer, stunted growth, reproductive system impairments, skin disorders such as acne, and slight damage to the liver.

7. Asbestos was a popular insulation material, but it was banned in the seventies due to its carcinogenic effects. Traces of asbestos can still be found in old homes that did not have their insulations replaced. Besides cancer, asbestos causes scarring on the lung tissue.

8. Toxic heavy metals such as lead, arsenic, and mercury can still be found in various objects such as cheaply-made toys, preserved wood, antiperspirants, and building materials. Once those metals are inhaled or ingested, they can cause cancer, brain and nerve disorders such as Alzheimer's disease, nausea, lesser amounts of red and white blood cells, and abnormal heartbeats.

9. Chloroform is a common chemical that is used to make other chemicals. It is prevalent in the air, in water, and in food. It can cause cancer, infertility, birth defects, headaches, dizziness, and damage to the liver and kidneys.

10. Chlorine is commonly found in water as it is used to purify it. Whether from the typical drinking water or from a swimming pool, too much of chlorine will cause all sorts of respiratory problems such as sore throat, accumulation of fluid in the lungs, and asthma.

Based on this list, many of those toxins in the environment are brought about by humanity's modern lifestyles. Before they do undue harm to the body, especially the dreaded cancer, they must be flushed out promptly.

Other Sources of Toxins

Besides the ten most common toxic substances, there are also other toxins that can be found in almost everything in the modern world. It is inevitable that one must intake those toxins unknowingly, one way or the other.

The two most popular vices, which are smoking and drinking, are the other major reasons for the body's toxicity. Both alcohol and nicotine have been proven many times by the scientific community to be not just toxic, but also addicting. Those two substances also alter the brain's functions. Other toxic substances include caffeine, empty sugars, and saturated fats. The latter two are especially notorious for being fat fodder since they cannot be processed into needed energy.

Many cosmetics today also contain toxic substances such as VOCs that can be absorbed into the skin. Some cosmetics producers have already taken steps in ridding their beauty products of those toxins.

Taking too many medications all at once can also cause the body to be laced with toxins, since they are not properly eliminated from the body. If the body feels too taxed from a cornucopia of meds, a consultation with the doctor will help.

There are also naturally-occurring toxins that are used by certain plants and animals as defense mechanisms against invaders. Snakes and jellyfish have highly deadly toxins and should not be consumed as food. A Japanese dish called *fugu* uses a type of blowfish that releases toxins which will certainly kill someone who eats an improperly-prepared version of the dish.

Processed foods, especially canned goods, are also a major source of toxins. While those foods contain preservatives that prolong their shelf lives, they unknowingly unleash a world of hurt on one who voraciously eats these. Needless to say, one must balance those foods out with naturally-grown foods.

Chapter 2: Why Must We Detoxify?

Detoxification is not just the simple flushing out of unwanted substances when the body cannot handle expelling them on its own. It is also the purging of impure thoughts in the mind that cause all sorts of decisions to inhale and ingest several toxins, whether knowingly or unknowingly, into the body. To ensure that an individual is rightfully clean in both body and mind, all sorts of unwanted things must be eliminated, especially in the detox diet.

The Body Does It Own Job...

The excretory system does its job of purging waste substances from the body via its two major processes: urination and release of excrement. Urination is obviously handled by the urinary system, while the release of excrement is handled by the lower parts of the digestive system.

The urinary system's main actor is the kidneys. The kidneys filter unwanted stuff such as ammonia, urea, uric acid, and excess salt and water from the blood as well as other bodily fluids. Those unwanted stuff then get to the bladder, which acts as a temporary storage. If the bladder gets full, the stuff gets expelled out of the urethra in the form of urine. Ammonia is a byproduct of the breakdown and usage of protein for the body's energy, while urea and uric acid are less toxic substances that result from the breakdown of ammonia.

The lower parts of the digestive system consist of the liver, the intestines, and the colon. The liver does its job of breaking down foreign substances so that the kidneys can have an easier job filtering them out as urine. The intestines and the colon facilitate the expelling of solid waste substances in the form of feces. The colon, in particular, absorbs trace minerals such as potassium and sends them to the bloodstream before they are included as feces that will be expelled by pooping.

Another natural detoxifier found in the human body is the lymphatic system. The lymphatic system contains lymph nodes that are scattered throughout the body but are interconnected. Those nodes provide the body with immunity, complementing the immune system, by filtering out unwelcome invaders such as bacteria, viruses, old red blood cells, and other toxic substances.

Other parts of the excretory system consist of the lungs and skin. The lungs expel excess water and carbon dioxide when someone breathes out. The skin kicks out excess water, salt, uric acid, and excess trace minerals in the form of sweat.

...But It Is Not Enough in the Modern Age

However, as demonstrated in the previous chapter, there are far too many substances that are deemed toxic in the wrong amounts. With humanity's modern lifestyles, the body does not know what to make of the increasing number of unwelcome invaders in its insides. These usually never get flushed out as urine and feces, but instead accumulate in the body fat.

As the invaders multiply and never get flushed out, they get in the way of the body's usual processes and will cause several problems such as depleted energy levels, unnatural weight gain, and various diseases that target the major body systems.

Another thing that is not helping the body in its natural detoxification process is the busy and hectic schedules people normally have. Because those people have no time to perform even mundane healthy tasks such as drinking adequate water, the body never gets its supply of natural detox assistants. Couple the lack of those assistants with stress and it will be a recipe for disaster.

Therefore, it is important that in this world of toxicity, people must amplify their bodily defenses against all sorts of foreign toxic substances by enhancing the many components of the excretory system such as the kidneys, the liver, the intestines, and the colon. With the contaminants out of the way, the body's natural healing processes also get their groove back. As the major organ systems work hand-in-hand, the benefits that are felt in one particular system will spread towards the other systems.

In short, steeling the body and its functions, especially the excretory functions, is one of the first lines of defense against toxin-induced sicknesses. There will be a marked loss in weight, since the excessive fats as well as the toxins they contain are properly expelled. There will also be renewed liveliness since the bodily functions that have something to do with the intake and processing of energy sources are no longer clogged by invasive toxins.

Why the Mind Is Also Important in Detoxification

The decisions a person makes, no matter how small they are, can contribute to huge consequences. For example, if one decides to commute to a bar, he or she gets all sorts of toxins in the process – airborne impurities from urban roads, food additives from the snacks he or she eats while commuting, nicotine and other chemicals from tobacco smoke generated by smokers inside and outside the bar, and alcohol from the hard drinks he or she consumes while in the bar.

Therefore, it is important that a person must think thoroughly and deeply before settling on a decision that will make him or her take in all those unwanted toxins along the way. Yes, this may turn him or her into a control freak, but there are also decisions that will endow him or her with long-term benefits. Remember, detoxification starts in the mind. The decisions that lead to the unknowing intake of toxins must be sorted out and eliminated from the usual routines first.

Chapter 3: The Crucial Ten Days

There are several forms of detoxification, and they more often than not involve ingesting special liquids and solids, cleansing the colon, foot baths and foot pads, spas and saunas, and fasting. But they also cost money, are always focused on the short-term effects, and may not deliver the detoxification results one desires. The best form of the detox diet must involve getting rid of major sources of toxins, ingesting more of the substances that will greatly assist the body's natural detoxification processes, never integrating any form of starvation or elimination of a major food group from the diet, and clearing the mind of impure thoughts that lead to impure actions. This way, the diet will grant long-term effects of well-being. As a beneficial consequence, this diet will cost little to no money, except for the money to be spent on detoxifying foods and drinks.

The ten days this detox diet contains are important to ensure natural weight loss and general well-being. And even after the diet period ends, some good habits contained in this diet, particularly the continued eating of healthy foods, must still be kept. This is to ensure that the person undergoing this diet will transition into a healthy lifestyle.

Preparing for the Diet

One important thing to do when undergoing this diet, or any other diet for that matter, is to not rush in immediately. A crash diet will have nasty consequences such as abrupt changing of body patterns that lead to all sorts of ailments as well as retention of the weight one lost during the diet routine. Therefore, one must start slow and transition into the diet carefully.

Not rushing in also applies to the chewing of food. The body needs some time to digest the food. Never treat the ten days of the diet like some kind of work deadline.

The usual vice-based sources of toxins, which are tobacco and alcohol, must be eliminated first. While dealing with the withdrawal effects of both of those substances may be difficult, timely help from a doctor who has a specialization in several types of addictions and substance abuse will lessen the difficulty.

In the three days before the actual start of the diet, rid the pantry and fridge of tempting foodstuffs that are loaded with empty calories. These include sweets and most forms of processed foods and fast food. At the same time, steadily increase the intake of fruits and vegetables – *especially organic ones.* As much as possible, turn the veggies into freshly-prepared salads and/or lightly steam them. As for the fruits, eat them raw and/or turn them into natural juices.

Since pesticide residue in fruits and vegetables is inevitable, the use of fruit and vegetable washes must be prioritized.

The intake of caffeine must be slowly and surely reduced to prevent withdrawal symptoms such as headaches. Switching to decaf coffee and low-caffeine teas such as green tea will help, as is the trick of diluting regular coffee and tea in huge amounts of water.

And speaking of water, the time-tested advice of eight to ten glasses of water a day will especially help the detox diet become successful. Drink it throughout the ten days of the diet.

Aromatherapy using essential oils is helpful, as this therapy helps to calm the mind in order for it to prepare for the rigors of the critical ten days.

Finally, before embarking on the detox diet itself, please consult a registered dietician who can recommend the detoxifying foods to be eaten based on your genetic makeup. Furthermore, *do not stop* taking prescribed medicine, as discontinuing medications can have devastating effects on the body. Diets are not meant to be one-man shows, especially if the individual still has to learn much about the intricacies of diet programs like this.

Eat and Drink Them

With the transition phase over, it is time to actually start the detox diet. Here is a comprehensive list of foods and drinks that must be ingested during the ten crucial days of the diet.

1. Organic fruits and vegetables are the main focus of the detox diet. It does not matter what the size or type of fruit or vegetable one will be consuming – as long as it is free of pesticides and synthetic fertilizers and is grown using age-old farming techniques, it certainly counts. Eat a good variety of fruits and vegetables to round out all the necessary nutrients.

2. Brown rice is much healthier compared to the typical white rice. As white rice is a result of the milling process, brown rice retains some nutrients that are usually lost during milling. This type of rice is also a rich source of fiber, which will aid in flushing the toxins out via the intestines and the colon.

3. Herbs are permissible, since they are also plants. Use them to flavor the dishes as well as utilize them for aromatherapy. Herbal teas are also a-OK, since they do not contain caffeine at all. As with fruits and vegetables, herbs must not have traces of anything toxic.

4. Whole-grain products, much like brown rice, do not undergo the nutrient-losing milling process. They are also rich sources of fiber. Whole-grain products include whole wheat bread, bran, and rolled oats.

5. Seaweeds such as kelp and *nori* wrappers used for sushi are also plant-based. They can also be consumed the same way as typical veggies do.

6. Beans such as green peas, chick peas, lentils, kidney beans, and black beans are permitted.

7. One can go nuts with nuts and seeds. Allowable things include almonds, cashews, walnuts, watermelon seeds, pumpkin

13

seeds, sunflower seeds, and sesame seeds. As a general rule, pick only raw, unsalted nuts and seeds.

8. Coconuts, while they are not actually nuts, are also allowed. There are several coconut-based consumables such as coconut water and coconut oil. One can also eat fresh coconut meat straight from the source.

9. Plant-based oils are encouraged. Olive oil, especially the extra virgin kind, is highly recommended.

10. Round out the protein-based nutrition with plant-based protein sources such as soy. Soy milk and tofu are easily-acquired sources of plant-based protein.

11. All sorts of edible mushrooms are permitted. Portobello and shiitake mushrooms can act as good substitutes for meat.

12. Natural sweeteners such as raw honey and natural maple syrup are permitted.

13. Besides herbs, other natural condiments that are tolerable include apple cider vinegar, sea salt, and mustard.

14. If there is still a desire to eat meat and get adequate protein, go with lean meats such as fish and organic chicken. Eggs are also on the list, as long as they are organic.

Never Eat and Drink Them

Meanwhile, these are the foods and drinks to avoid during the detox diet phase.

1. In general, non-lean types of red meat are off-limits. Canned meat is especially forbidden.

2. All forms of processed foods containing all sorts of additives and preservatives are out of the question. On a related note, artificial sweeteners and processed condiments are also out.

3. Typical white sugar and brown sugar are verboten, as well as high-fructose syrups.

4. Corn must be avoided as it is acid-forming. The acid in question is uric acid. Furthermore, the corn kernels that are indigestible will make bathroom breaks more excruciating.

5. While nuts are OK, peanuts and peanut butter are usually excluded.

6. Milk is normally not allowed, but half a cup of yogurt containing good bacteria per day is an exception to that.

7. Caffeine is another typical forbidden substance.

8. Shortening and margarine are inadmissible.

9. While fish is OK, other seafoods are not.

Other Cleansing Procedures

There are many variations of the detox diet, but the one being presented in this book will not involve complicated doohickeys and specialized food and drinks to amplify the detoxification effect. Here are some things one can also do during the ten days of the diet.

With all the conveniences of Internet-based connectivity, sometimes too much is too much. Dedicate one of the ten days, or even all ten days, to a temporary break from technology. Put away the smartphone or tablet, avoid touching the computer, and never be tempted to go online just about anywhere. Take the time off from technology to visit someplace serene, like a retreat house. This technology break will clear the mind of all sorts of burdening thoughts that may poison one's thinking the same way that bodily toxins do.

Take some time off to scrape the tongue. Tongue scraping is a practice in ayurvedic medicine, or ancient Hindu medicine, where all the impurities built up on the tongue are removed. Tongue scrapers can be bought for cheap at drug store.

Try to write all the stored thoughts and feelings, even negative ones, into a diary or notebook. Releasing all the stored strong emotions to a diary or notebook has a cathartic effect, since keeping those emotions locked away will eventually take the toll on one's health.

Another mind-cleansing procedure one can do during the ten days is meditation. Meditation also helps clear the mind of toxic thoughts that lead to stress, which then slows down the liver's detoxification process. Yoga is especially helpful as a meditation tool. You may also augment your meditation by doing deep breathing exercises or visualizing relaxing images such as watching the sunset at the beach.

Get enough dosages of vitamin C. While the vitamin is better known for boosting immunity, it also helps the body with the production of glutathione. Glutathione may be better known as a skin rejuvenating agent, but it also exists in the liver as a detoxification aid. Citrus fruits are the best-known sources of vitamin C.

Enhance blood circulation, since poor blood circulation will hamper the flushing out of impurities from the blood. Exercise is a guaranteed way to get that blood pumping.

Keep in mind that not all bacteria are bad. Good bacteria mostly reside in the intestines, aiding in digestion and preventing bad bacteria from releasing toxins that can be deployed in the bloodstream. Help the good bacteria by taking probiotic drinks.

Chapter 4: Detoxification Recipes

Breakfast Recipes

Gut-Busting Oatmeal Bowl

Ingredients:

- 1-2 cups oatmeal

- 1-2 cups water or nut milk

- A mixture of fresh berries and fresh fruits, all sliced

Procedure:

1. Prepare the oatmeal as indicated in the packaging.

2. While hot, pour the berries and fruits onto the prepared oatmeal, and mix.

Berry Blast Smoothie

Ingredients:

- 1-2 cups mixed fresh berries
- 1-2 cups protein powder
- 1-2 cups ice cubes

Procedure:

1. Throw all the ingredients into a blender, and hit puree.
2. Serve the smoothie in a tall glass.

Lunch Recipes

Veggie Cavalcade Salad with Tofu

Ingredients:

- 6-8 pieces of any whole vegetable (for greens, an amount of at least five leaves equals one whole piece)

- 1-2 pieces tofu, diced

- 4-5 teaspoons extra virgin olive oil

- 2 teaspoons fresh lemon juice

- 1 teaspoon freshly-chopped herbs of choice

Procedure:

1. Fry the tofu in 2-3 teaspoons olive oil until slightly browned. Set aside.

2. Slice and/or dice the vegetables into reasonably-sized pieces. Leave the greens untouched.

3. Pour all the vegetables and the tofu into a bowl. Mix completely.

4. Combine 2 teaspoons olive oil, the lemon juice, and the herbs to make the dressing.

5. Pour the dressing all over the salad. Mix completely.

Special Omelet Rice

Ingredients:

- 3-5 organic eggs
- Fresh or dried herbs (any variety), to taste
- 2-3 teaspoons extra virgin olive oil
- 1-2 cups cooked brown rice

Procedure:

1. Beat the eggs into a scramble while adding the herbs.

2. Pour the olive oil into a heated pan. Wait until the oil is hot.

3. Pour the egg and herb mixture until the omelet is formed. Turn over to ensure proper cooking.

4. Once the omelet is out of the pan, place the brown rice inside it. Make sure the omelet wraps around the rice.

5. Serve hot with mustard.

Dinner Recipes

The Steamed Medley

Ingredients:

- 1 slice salmon

- 5-10 pieces broccoli and asparagus (can be of any combination)

- 1/4 cup fresh lemon juice

- Fresh or dried herbs (any variety), to taste

Procedure:

1. In a steamer or a rice cooker with a steaming basket, arrange the salmon slice and the broccoli and asparagus pieces so that the steam will be evenly distributed.

2. Sprinkle the salmon and the vegetables with the lemon juice and fresh herbs.

3. Begin steaming the salmon and the vegetables. Seven to ten minutes is enough for the lemon and the herbs to seep into the steamed content.

4. Serve hot.

Glorified Bunch of Small Potatoes

Ingredients:

- 6 ounces small potatoes
- 4 tablespoons extra virgin olive oil
- Any natural condiment of choice

Procedure:

1. Gently simmer the potatoes in water for 5-10 minutes. Drain them off afterwards. Retain the peels beforehand.

2. Heat the olive oil in a roasting tin, but not to burning levels.

3. Roast every side of the potatoes until crisp and golden brown. This will take at most 45 minutes.

4. Serve hot with the condiment of choice.

Snack and Drink Recipes

Veggie Brown Rice Sushi

Ingredients:

- 1 cup cooked brown rice

- 1 *nori* wrapper

- Any sliced or diced vegetable that can fit inside the sushi

Procedure:

1. Mold the brown rice into any shape, whether in a tube form or rolled into a ball. The important thing is that the vegetable must fit inside the sushi.

2. Wrap the *nori* wrapper around the formed brown rice.

3. Repeat steps 1 and 2 for any remaining amounts of vegetables, brown rice, and the *nori* wrapper.

Stretched Herbal Iced Tea

Ingredients:

- 1 bag herbal tea (any kind)
- 1 citrus fruit of choice (e.g. lemon or orange)
- 1 cup briskly-boiled water
- 2-3 cups lukewarm water
- Several ice cubes
- Honey, to taste

Procedure:

1. Depending on the strength of the resultant tea, submerge one teabag into briskly-boiled water.

2. Meanwhile, cut the citrus fruit of choice into slices that can be fit inside a glass.

3. Place the fruit slices into a tall glass that can accommodate at least five cups.

4. Carefully pour both the brewed tea and the lukewarm water into the tall glass at a distance of at least 12 inches from the glass. This is where the "stretched" part comes from, and one must avoid spills during the stretching process.

5. Add some dollops of honey based on the preferred amount of sweetness.

6. Finally, add the ice cubes.

Fruity Shaved Ice

Ingredients:

- 1-2 cups shaved ice

- 1/2-1 cup natural unsweetened fruit juice of any kind

Procedure:

1. Place the shaved ice in either a wide glass or a bowl.

2. Pour the unsweetened fruit juice on top of the shaved ice, and enjoy.

Note: One can replace shaved ice with shaved or crushed frozen fruit.

Chapter 5: Some Friendly Reminders

As with every other diet program on the planet, care, precise planning, patience, and perseverance must be taken to heart when undergoing the detoxification diet. Even in a short period like ten days, many things will happen. To ensure that the detox diet will become a success that will beget many more successes in the realm of the healthy lifestyle, keep the following friendly reminders in mind.

Do Not Starve

Other detox diets recommend taking only the formulas they sell themselves. Indeed, they may contain needed plant-based nourishment needed for detoxification, but the makers of those diets often forget that an imbalanced diet that is lacking in calories will prove detrimental to the body. Not only will the energy levels be depleted, but the metabolism process will also be slowed down. One unpleasant aftereffect is the tendency to eat more, especially unhealthy foods, once the diet period is over. This will make natural weight loss almost unachievable. Even worse, the lack of micronutrients in these other detox diets will lead to malnutrition that is based on micronutrient deficiency, which opens yet another floodgate of diseases. Other nasty effects of other detox crash diets include muscle degeneration, since the muscles have no source of energy to turn to, and an imbalance in blood sugar levels.

Hence, this detox diet espouses the idea that *forced starvation is absolutely prohibited*. Just eat the recommended foods at will and in good, moderated amounts.

Expect to Pee (and Poop and Sweat) a Lot

Since the detox diet enhances the body's natural detox functions, expect one undergoing the diet to pee a lot. Water, in particular, helps in flushing out toxins.

Excessive peeing not just happens when the detox diet goes overboard. Excessive sweating also happens, as well as the resultant excrement being too liquid and nasty-smelling. Peeing, pooping, and sweating too much can lead to dehydration if the amount of fluids being taken is not immediately replenished.

Dehydration is not just the depletion of the body's water, but is also the disrupted balance of fluids and electrolytes that can lead to ailments such as gastrointestinal distress, headaches, fatigue, irritability, skin irritations, circulatory problems, kidney failure, and heat stroke. Death also awaits one who is severely dehydrated.

To counteract dehydration, do not depend on fluids and fluids alone, unlike what some detox diets emphasize. Be well-balanced in both solids and liquids to avoid lost hours as a result of abnormally frequent trips to the bathroom.

Want a Colonic? No Thanks

Another form of the detox therapy involves cleansing the colon and intestines of toxins that may be released into the bloodstream. However, as demonstrated in the third chapter, there are beneficial bacteria that reside in the colon and intestines. If those bacteria are flushed out, the normal digestive process will be hampered, and the bad bacteria will have a good time releasing more toxins since their rivals are gone. The flushing out of good bacteria also results from the detox diet going beyond the recommended ten days.

Another bad effect of colon cleansing is dehydration, for the same reasons demonstrated in the previous section. Trace minerals such as potassium are also lost during the cleansing process, which contributes to dehydration. Other side effects of colon cleansing include nausea and vomiting.

Diet as an End to the Means, Not a Means to the End

People who want the figures of their dreams often forget that dieting is not really meant to immediately shed unwanted pounds. Dieting is truly meant for improved nourishment and nutrition. The notions of shedding that slab or beer belly in preparation for an event like showing off in a bikini should be disposed of. A proper mindset must be established first when doing the detox diet or any other diet for that matter.

As stated before, the detox diet being demonstrated in this book should be a transitional phase to a healthier lifestyle. Thinking in the long term when dieting is certainly better than thinking in the short term. One should remember that dieting must be an end to unhealthy habits and not a means to end that "awful" figure.

Conclusion

Thank you again for purchasing *"Detox Diet Guide: Lose Weight Quickly, Achieve Optimal Health and Feel Energized Through the 10 Day Detox"*!

I hope this book was able to help you to understand the ins and outs of the detox diet and why it is important to achieve a major change in only a short time.

Are you ready for the change? Tony Robbins says in order to create effective change, you need to start by being disgusted with where you are at. Are you disgusted with your health or body? Is it an ABSOLUTE MUST to change...not another moment? You need to feel the pain of where you are at to get the urgency to change and manifest the momentum to take action.

The next step is to consult your doctor or dietician before embarking on such a diet. And once you are given the final OK, you can then consult various more detoxification recipes based on the comprehensive list of allowable foods and drinks in this book. The recipes given in this book is just a starting point.

Finally, if you enjoyed this book, please take the time to share your thoughts and post a review on Amazon. It would be greatly appreciated!

I would love for you to share your experiences, stories and encouragements with me. My email address is

emmarosekindle@gmail.com

In addition, please remember to check out our Facebook page in order to find other resources and upcoming promotions:

https://www.facebook.com/joypublishing

With sincere thanks,

Emma Rose

Preview of "Clean Eating Guide: Lose Weight Quickly, Achieve Optimal Health and Feel Energized with Clean Eating for Busy Families and Clean Eating Recipes

Introduction

I want to thank you and congratulate you for purchasing the book, *"Clean Eating Guide: Lose Weight Quickly, Achieve Optimal Health and Feel Energized with Clean Eating For Busy Families and Clean Eating Recipes"*.

This book contains proven steps and strategies on how to lose weight, have more energy, and stay healthy using the principles of clean eating.

There are so many different kinds of diet programs and products available in the market today and all you need to do is choose the one that you think will work best for you. If you do not want to try new products that helps you lose weight and boosts your energy, you should stick to something more basic and natural such as clean eating.

In this book, you will learn everything you need to know about clean eating. It is important to find out everything you can about this type of diet before you incorporate it in your lifestyle. You will learn about the benefits and principles of clean eating and some useful tips that can help you along the way. This book also includes some easy recipes that promote clean eating.

Thanks again for purchasing this book, I hope you enjoy it! Please take some time to stop by and LIKE our Facebook page:

https://www.facebook.com/joypublishing

With gratitude,

Emma Rose

Chapter 1

What Is Clean Eating?

You have probably come across the term 'clean eating' but you are still not familiar about its exact meaning. This is being used by people who work in the health and fitness industry such as personal trainers ad dietitians. People who are health conscious and workout fanatic also often use this word. Does it have something to do with cleaning the food before eating or cooking? Or maybe it has something to do with the kind of food that you eat.

The loose definition of clean eating is eating food in its most natural state. These days, people are starting to pay more attention to the kinds of food that they eat and how these foods are made. They take note of the food's ingredients and make sure that the food product only contains all natural ingredients.

The term clean eating first came out in the 1990s. Today, it is still being used by health conscious individuals from different backgrounds and culture to refer to the kind of all natural diet that they have. The definition of clean eating can vary from person to person. Some define clean eating as eating mostly fruits and vegetables while others define it as not eating anything artificial. You will find out more about these things as you read this book.

What Clean Eating is not?

If you think clean eating is another diet program, like the South Beach diet or Paleo diet, you are wrong because clean eating is a way of life. It also does not follow any strict rules about what food group to eat and not to eat, how many calories you should consume in a meal, and so on. This is the most basic way of healthy eating that promotes weight loss and boost energy. Everybody can do this, even those who are not trying to lose weight.

Clean eating will not make you feel deprived or frustrated because it is so easy to follow. You do not even need to have a really strong determination because it is all a matter of choosing natural over artificial.

Is there such a thing as 'dirty' eating?

You are probably wondering if there is such a thing as 'dirty' eating or the opposite of clean eating. Clean eating does not literally mean eating foods that have less dirt. It means that you are choosing the best and healthiest food choices from different food groups in their most natural state. 'Dirty' eating is not the opposite of clean eating because there is no such thing as eating dirty. The opposite of clean eating is choosing the wrong food to eat and eating junk foods and processed foods that leave toxins in your body.

Clean eating also looks at the source of food. It should not come from large commercial manufacturers that use machines to process food. The foods that clean eaters usually use come from small farms that do not use chemicals and undergo processes. This is why clean eating is often associated with organic eating.

Check out the rest of "Clean Eating Guide: Lose Weight Quickly. Achieve Optimal Health and Feel Energized with Clean Eating for Busy Families and Clean Eating Recipes" on Amazon.

Check Out My Other Books

Below you'll find some of my other books also available on Amazon and Kindle. Search for these titles on the Amazon website to find them.

Paleo Free Diet Guide for Beginners: Over 50 Paleo Free Recipes for Optimal Health & Fast Weight Loss

Paleo Desserts: Satisfy Your Sweet Tooth With Over 100 Quick & Easy Paleo Dessert Recipes & Paleo Baking Recipes

Raw Food Diet Guide: Lose Weight Quickly, Achieve Optimal Health & Feel Energized with the Raw Food Diet & Raw Food Recipes

Clean Eating Guide: Lose Weight Quickly, Achieve Optimal Health & Feel Energized with Clean Eating For Busy Families & Clean Eating Recipes

Alkaline Diet Guide: Lose Weight Quickly, Achieve Optimal Health & Feel Energized with the Alkaline Diet & Alkaline Recipes

Coconut Flour Recipes for Optimal Health & Quick Weight Loss: Gluten Free Recipes for Celiac Disease, Gluten Sensitivities & Paleo Free Diets

Almond Flour Recipes for Optimal Health & Quick Weight Loss: Gluten Free Recipes for Celiac Disease, Gluten Sensitivities & Paleo Free Diets

Wheat Free Diet for Beginners: Lose Weight Quickly, Achieve Optimal Health & Feel Energized with Gluten Free Recipes for Celiac Disease, Gluten Sensitivities & Paleo Free Diets

Detox Diet Guide: Lose Weight Quickly, Achieve Optimal Health & Feel Energized Through the 10 Day Detox

Sugar Detox Guide for Beginners: Lose Weight Quickly, Achieve Optimal Health, Feel Energized & Eliminate Sugar Cravings Naturally

Ketogenic Diet Guide for Beginners: How to Achieve Rapid Weight Loss, Optimal Health & Unstoppable Energy with Ketogenic Diet Recipes

Anti Inflammatory Diet for Beginners: Lose Weight Fast, Optimize Health, Slow Aging, Fight Inflammation, Conquer Pain & Increase Energy with the Anti Inflammation Diet Recipes

One Last Thing...

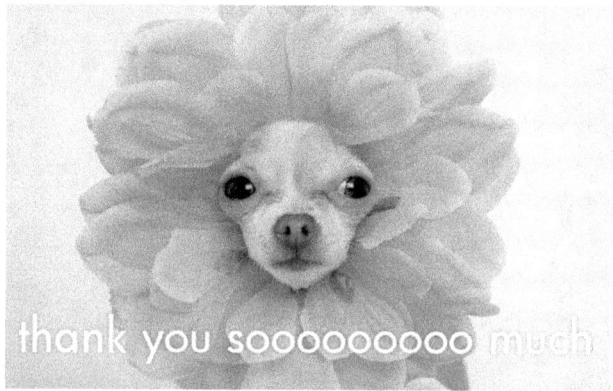

Source: Wikipedia

If you believe that this book is worth sharing, would you please take the time to let others know how it affected your life? If it turns out to make a difference in the lives of others, they will be forever grateful to you, as will I.

www.ingramcontent.com/pod-product-compliance
Lightning Source LLC
Chambersburg PA
CBHW060109300526
45791CB00018B/505